INTERMITTENT FASTING

LOSE WEIGHT, HEAL YOUR BODY, AND LIVE A HEALTHY LIFE!

Amanda Walker

TABLE OF CONTENTS

INTRODUCTION

Unless you've been in a coma for the past few decades, you're no doubt aware that there's a worrisome epidemic afflicting millions of people all over the globe. That epidemic is obesity, excessive weight that leads to physical and mental health problems that affect quality of life. The latest buzz is about "belly fat" which is the term that has been coined to describe abdominal obesity. The common occurrence of this phenomenon is clearly evident to the most casual observer on a bus or in the shopping mall. In fact, the words "belly fat" have become a sort of battle cry of health professionals and nutritionists who recognize the dangers lurking behind all that fat.

Excess weight in general, and belly fat in particular, have all sorts of negative effects on your body, your heart, and even your brain. Increased weight means an increased risk of developing heart problems, type 2 diabetes, inflammatory diseases, and cancer. Looking at the big picture, a larger waist circumference can lead to a shorter life. As much as we try to fool ourselves with lame excuses, the principal cause of this problem is pretty clear: We eat too much.

But it's more than that. Many of the foods we eat are poor sources of nutrients. In our quest for foods that are convenient and tasty, we often forgo the right kinds of foods that we need for a healthy life. We have become a society that tends to eat whatever we want, whenever we want, wherever we can get it. Then one day something happens: We step on the scale, or we see our reflection in a mirror, or we can't get our jeans up past our thighs, and we think, "Oh, ___!" [Choose your favorite expletive.]

It's time to do something, and the first thing that comes to mind is the D word--diet. But now there's another problem. In the late 1970s the USDA recommended a low fat diet, and that seems to be just about the point at which the rate of obesity began its statistical climb. In cutting down on fats, people began to consume more carbohydrates, which stimulate insulin levels. High insulin levels actually make people gain weight, rather than losing it. That was the opposite of what the USDA intended.

When the recommended low-fat diet didn't produce the desired results, more diets began to come out of the woodwork. We went from low-fat to low-carb, to slow-carb, Atkins, South Beach, Zone, Mediterranean, all liquid, all vegetable, all fruit, all raw, and so on, and so on. Companies like Jenny Craig and Nutrisystem also jumped on the diet bandwagon, and Slimfast and Ayds developed products to help in the weight loss effort.

The results were mixed. Many of these diets were successful with a lot of people, but many were not. That's the thing about dieting: What works for one person won't work for another. Finding a diet that's perfect for everybody has just not been accomplished at this point. That's why diet books continue to be hot items in bookstores and libraries everywhere.

One refrain that seems to prevail among all the diets is the question, "What can I eat today?" With all the calorie counting, fat counting, carb counting, etc., we often find that our daily choices are limited. But what if there were some days where, instead of saying, "What can I eat today?" you could say, "What will I eat today?"

It's not just wishful thinking that you would be able to eat whatever you liked on a diet. With intermittent fasting, it's a reality. That doesn't mean that you'll be wolfing down giant portions of ice cream and french fries at will. With intermittent fasting, there will still be some restrictions. The difference is that you will not be restricting *what* you eat, but *when* you eat. And not only will you lose weight, you'll also become healthier in the process.

PART 1: WHAT IS

INTERMITTENT FASTING?

WHAT IS INTERMITTENT FASTING, AND WHY IS IT GOOD FOR YOU?

By definition, intermittent fasting (IF) means that a person has regularly scheduled periods of time where she eats a normal diet, alternating with periods of restricted eating. In other words, it's a pattern of skipping meals on a regular basis. Restricted eating could be anything from zero calories to a small quantity of food with a significantly minimized calorie total. For some people, it's a more effective way to lose weight than the other diet plans. At first, it's not easy--the hunger pangs during the fasting periods are impossible to ignore, and there's a constant need to watch the clock. But after a brief period of adjustment, the hunger pangs become insignificant, and the routine of intermittent fasting begins to fit right into the daily groove.

Some people will balk at the idea of not being able to indulge in their three to six meals a day, but if you think about it, you're already fasting every time you sleep. That's why the first meal of the day is called "breakfast"--you're "breaking" the "fast" between the last meal of yesterday and the first meal of today. So how hard can it be to just fast a bit longer, and wait a while for that first meal? Once your body gets adjusted to fasting on a regular timetable, your insulin and glucose levels will calm down (more on this later), and your brain won't be sending as many false alarms that you *need* to eat. The longer you maintain a regular fasting pattern, the easier it becomes.

One problem with our eating habits is just that: They are based on *habit.* Breakfast at 7:30 AM, lunch at noon on the dot, snacks at 10:00 and 3:00, and dinner at 6:00 with ice cream in front of the TV. And don't forget the requisite guacamole and chips while you watch football. All this whether you're hungry or not.

With intermittent fasting, you become more aware of your hunger levels. If there are certain times or circumstances where you eat because that's what you've always done, being on a fast means that you won't eat during those times, and eventually it will lead you to wonder why it was always such a big deal in the first place.

With intermittent fasting, your attitude toward eating becomes more purposeful, and you become more focused on your eating patterns. Once your attention is centered more on when you will eat than what you can eat, you no longer have to be as concerned with trying to eat less. As long as you don't try to overcompensate by bingeing between fasts, your average calorie count will naturally decrease, and you'll lose weight.

The idea of intermittent fasting as a weight loss/health improvement diet program is relatively new; for that reason, there has not been a lot of research done to verify all the anecdotal evidence from people who have tried it and are impressed with the results. According to some, the weight loss and loss of belly fat was remarkable. Not only that, but compared to eating a low calorie diet with no fasting period, the weight loss is just as effective, and possibly even more effective, but there is less muscle loss.

Is IF a good idea for everyone? Unfortunately, no. For people with certain health conditions, diabetes or malnutrition, for example, intermittent fasting could mean a serious risk to their health. And people with eating disorders would only aggravate their condition if they adopted the practice of intermittent fasting. Additionally, children, as well as women who are pregnant or breastfeeding, should not have nutritional restrictions. And before you make the decision whether intermittent fasting is for you, it's important to take into consideration any prescription meds that you take on a regular basis. If you happen to be on a medication that needs to be taken with food, fasting won't work for you. So the bottom line here is the same as with any type of diet: Do not proceed until you check all the facts and get the go-ahead from your health care provider.

The right mindset is very important for anyone who wishes to succeed with an intermittent fasting lifestyle. If you have a casual attitude toward it, it won't work for you. You're going to have to commit yourself to spending time on meal planning and preparation. Your social life will also factor in because so much of our interpersonal lives include a good amount of eating and drinking with friends and family. And if you're the type of person who starts feeling obsessive about food at the first sign of hunger pangs, this style of eating will probably make you miserable and more than a little bit crazy. When you are constantly thinking about food, you often tend to overcompensate for fasting by taking the first opportunity and eating more calories than you normally would. If that's the case, intermittent fasting may turn out to be more harmful than beneficial.

But for most people, there is some form of intermittent fasting that will fit in well with their needs and lifestyle and that they can be comfortable with over a long period. Later in this book, we will be discussing the many different eating/fasting methods that fall under the category of internet fasting.

A BRIEF HISTORY OF FASTING

Before you protest that fasting is unnatural and unhealthy, stop and think about our very first ancestors, the hunter-gatherers. Their very way of life subjected them to periods of imposed fasting because there were plenty of times when there was very little to hunt or gather. They probably had ways of making their available food stretch out over a longer period of time, but ultimately they had to become accustomed to eating when there was food available, and fasting when it was hard to find. It must have worked for them, somehow, because we're still here.

Then, during the first agricultural revolution, humans developed some know-how so that they could have some control over the availability of food. They domesticated and raised animals for meat, eggs, and milk, and they cultivated land and planted crops so that they would have reliable sources of food. This transition to agriculture also created a new lifestyle; since they no longer had to live a nomadic lifestyle to find food, our ancestors established settlements and stopped moving around. This gave them the opportunity to direct their focus to something beside their survival, and they began to think.

That brings us to the early philosophers. Pythagoras, Plutarch, Plato, Socrates, Aristotle, and other great thinkers and healers were all advocates of the practice of fasting. They believed in the power of fasting to clarify the mind and revitalize the body. Hippocrates, the father of medicine as a science, believed that fasting was an effective component of the healing process. He claimed, among other things, that, "When the patient is fed too richly, the disease is fed as well." Benjamin Franklin, a more modern thinker, claimed that, "The best of all medicines is resting and fasting."

When you think about it, fasting when you're sick makes a lot of sense. We actually possess a sort of fasting instinct. Your pets are a good example; when an animal doesn't feel well, it won't eat. And you can probably relate to the idea yourself. Think about the last time you had a bad case of the flu, and the thought of eating anything was revolting. That's because your body needed to direct as many of its resources as possible to fighting the illness, and working on the digestive process after eating would take some of those resources away. So fasting is the body's natural prescription to help you get well.

During the twentieth century, a number of therapeutic fasting clinics and centers popped up in some countries. These clinics generally specialized in certain types of fasts, such as water fasts or juice fasts, with medical supervision. Limotherapy, which involves abstaining from food for a period of one to one and a half days under medical supervision, became a popular method of therapeutic fasting at many of these clinics. Some of them even promoted their therapies as "fasting holidays." As trends change, these clinics continue to come and go.

Another modern trend in fasting has been cleansing fasts, which have become a popular way to detoxify the body. By abstaining from food and drinking only water, your system flushes out toxins that accumulate from food, pollution, and other contaminants that humans are constantly exposed to. Besides the water fast, there are a variety of other cleansing fasts that promote drinking juice, adding apple cider vinegar or lemon to the water, green smoothies, and more.

Fasting also has a long history in religion. Most religions today observe periods of time when followers are encouraged (or required) to show their commitment, faith, and spirituality by refraining from the indulgence of eating. In the case of religious fasting, practitioners feel that fasting is a good thing for both body and spirit. It's believed that fasting is a type of sacrifice that indicates purification and devoutness. Many religions turn to fasting in times of mourning and as a demonstration of penance. Many Christians fast for forty days during Lent because Christ fasted for forty days in the wilderness.

The prophet of Islam, Muhammad, was also devoted to fasting, so Muslims are expected to observe the holy month of Ramadan by eating and drinking nothing at all between sunrise and sunset every day. If fasting would be risky for someone because of health or age issues, they are allowed to substitute generosity to the poor for fasting. Once the sun has set, however, fasting Muslims often overindulge to compensate for what they missed during their fast, so they don't acquire the health benefits.

Followers of Buddhism are also faithful believers in fasting. When the Buddha was a young man seeking enlightenment, he went through a period of self-denial so severe that he limited himself to eating a single grain of rice per day. He was close to death when he realized that he would have to be alive to achieve enlightenment, and that realization motivated him to adopt a more balanced routine of self-discipline and self-indulgence. Today's Buddhists practice fasting to achieve self-control and greater spirituality. Many Buddhist monks do not eat any solid food after noon every day, and some lay people do the same on days of the full moon.

The practice of yoga also recommends fasting for cleansing the body, spiritual renewal, and basic practicality. Avoiding food before a yoga practice ensures that the intestines will be clear, allowing for better access to certain postures. In addition, the digestion process competes with other body systems and organs for blood, which undermines the effect of the energy flow that yoga practice provides. Proponents of yogic fasting also assert that fasting increases flexibility.

Native American cultures have always been closely connected to nature and their bodies. They recognized the benefits of fasting and would include the practice in many of their sacred rituals and rites of passage. Fasting was also an important element in the Vision Quest. This ritual involved a solitary time in the wilderness, or, in some cases, a heated hut, or sweat lodge, where the person would fast to achieve a clear mind. The goal was to experience dreams or visions that suggested a solution to a problem or a certain direction to follow. In some cases, the vision was understood to be a message from a deity.

Nowadays, Vision Quests are not limited to Native American cultures but are available to mainstream people who are searching for something outside of their own modern experience. It's possible to find businesses who will set up a Vision Quest for any interested party,

Fasting has also been known to be an instrument for passive resistance and political protest, as in hunger strikes. One of the most well-known people to fast for political purposes was Mahatma Gandhi, who repeatedly went on hunger strikes to protest the oppression of India's poorest classes and Great Britain's dominance over India. The hoped-for result was to get public sympathy behind him and pressure the government to make changes in policy. On one fast, Gandhi fasted for a total of 21 days, drinking only water.

There have been other fasting protests in different parts of the world, as well. During the Suffragette movement in Great Britain, for instance, many women went on hunger strikes to draw attention to their crusade to allow women to vote. The government was not sympathetic, however, and the public was scandalized when some of the more influential women were imprisoned and force-fed in rather violent ways.

Over the centuries, there have clearly been both light sides and dark sides to fasting practices. In some cases, people have died because their enthusiasm for fasting overpowered their common sense. A woman named Dr. Linda Hazzard even used a fasting "clinic" as a venue for starving patients into health, but about a dozen of them didn't survive the treatment. Dr. Hazzard was ultimately tried for murder. Fortunately, cases like these are rare, but they emphasize the fact that there needs to be a sufficient amount of knowledge about the subject if one is to undertake fasting in any form.

COMMON MYTHS ABOUT FASTING

It's virtually impossible to show an interest in any diet or health program without becoming the recipient of other people's takes on the topic. If you're lucky, everyone you talk to will be a supporter and cheer you on throughout your journey. But if your circle of friends and acquaintances includes a skeptic or two, you're also likely hear about some of the myths that are linked to fasting. People tend to believe and repeat what they hear over and over again, so these myths have a tendency to never go away.

So, is a myth an outright lie, or is it a half-truth? It depends. In some cases, there is some sort of evidence that campaigners will claim "proves" the statement, but by taking these myths one by one and looking into the actual science, we can debunk the myths and follow human reason.

Myth number one: Fasting is a form of starvation.

This is true only in the sense that you do feel hungry, at first. Often, you feel very, very hungry, and many people would say, "I'm starving!" But technically, starvation means that you don't have sufficient food, and you don't see any prospects for food in the future. In other words, starvation is the restriction of calories without a choice. When you are fasting, you *choose* to restrict your calories for a specific period of time, and you know that there is an end to the fast and there will be food.

Some people are concerned that going on a fast will signal your body to move into "starvation mode" and shut down your metabolism so that you won't be burning the same number of calories. This is your body's defense against starvation when it recognizes that the number of calories being consumed has altered drastically. This does happen, but it happens when you cut down your calorie intake on any diet, not just IF. And it's not necessarily a bad thing.

Actually, there is evidence that shows that fasting for short periods, up to 48 hours, can actually speed up your metabolism because of an increase in hormones that break down body fat. However, fasting for longer than 48 hours can slow down the metabolism, so it seems to be all about timing.

The bottom line here is that anyone can go too far with a fast so that it has the potential to become a form of starvation. Gandhi and the Buddha are historical examples of this, and they came pretty close to dying. Examples like these are likely to have started this particular myth in the first place, but they are too extreme to be considered a viable reason for this myth to be taken at face value.

Myth number two: It's a good idea to eat frequent small meals throughout the day to regulate your metabolism and control hunger.

While it's true that your body does need some energy to digest food and carry all the nutrients to their proper places, it really depends on the total number of calories you consume during the day, not how many meals you eat. You will burn about ten percent of your total calorie consumption on digesting the food. The studies on eating habits of individuals concluded that it didn't matter how often they ate or how many meals they had. The results were the same for the people who ate several meals and those who ate fewer meals with the same number of calories.

Another reason that some people make the claim that it's better to eat several small meals through the day is the question of how the body uses protein. Proponents of frequent meals insist that the body needs to have protein every two or three hours to support the development of muscles. Scientific studies, however, don't support this claim. What matters is how much protein you have all together, not per meal.

Do frequent small meals help stave off hunger pangs? Studies on this question have come up yes, no, and maybe. This seems to be a question that depends on the varying physical and psychological traits that all humans possess.

Myth number three: Fasting deprives your brain of the glucose it needs to function.

Yes, the brain uses glucose, but it has other options if the glucose isn't immediately available. If you're not eating enough food to produce glucose, your body goes into defense mode and turns to the stored glycogen in the liver. If food is restricted for longer periods, as it is in fasting, the body turns to the ketone bodies that are produced when fatty acids are burned. Ketone bodies are a great source of fuel for the brain, but some people report having headaches during the early stages of fasting that seem to be related to the presence of ketone bodies. These headaches can be alleviated by drinking plenty of fluids.

Myth number four: You lose muscle when you fast.

This is mostly true, but it really depends on what type of fasting you're talking about. If you fast for an extended amount of time, a month or more, for example, your body will run out of fuel sources and start to seek out muscle. But this would be an act of desperation. Recent studies indicate that consuming muscle is a last resort, and it will only be consumed as fuel when the body has burned through its stores of glucose, then fat, then ketone bodies. When it does turn to protein, it will be unnecessary protein, such as skin tags, before it actually begins to metabolize muscle.

Intermittent fasting up to three or four days in duration is perfectly safe for everyone who is in good health, according to Dr. Jason Fung, creator of the 5:2 intermittent fast. In fact, a study where participants consumed all their calories in one meal showed that their muscle mass actually increased. That's most likely due to the fact that intermittent fasting causes an increase in growth hormones.

Whatever weight loss method you follow, you can reduce the chances of muscle loss by making sure you are getting sufficient protein when you are eating and to include a weight-based exercise program in your routine.

Myth number five: Intermittent fasting is harmful to your health.

Some people believe that fasting deprives your body of vital nutrients you need to keep you healthy. Again, this can be true if you take it too far. But there is plenty of anecdotal evidence and a fair number of scientific studies that show that intermittent fasting actually provides a number of benefits for your health. These benefits include protection against some diseases, greater longevity of life, reduced inflammation, and improved brain function. More on benefits in the next section.

Myth number six: Intermittent fasting will actually make you gain weight because you'll get so hungry that you will overeat when you're not fasting.

This is another half-truth, but again, it depends on individual behavior. For most people, resuming a normal diet, with perhaps a few extra calories, will not undo the good you did while fasting. However, if you *over*compensate for the meals you missed, of course you will be consuming too many calories for weight loss. As long as you have the proper mindset, you will realize that your hunger can be controlled with moderate amounts of nutritious food. In addition, personal experience of many people on a fasting regimen has shown that appetite actually tends to diminish as the fasting continues. As long as the non-fasting calories stay below the calories missed while fasting, you will lose weight.

BENEFITS OF FASTING

Unless you have an illness, any type of weight loss is going to affect your body and your health in a positive way. So what makes fasting different? It's the way your body responds. Because of your body's natural defense mechanisms to a lack of nourishment, it will adapt to the situation by producing enzymes and hormones that provide a range of benefits. This doesn't happen if you are just "cutting down" on calories, fats, or carbs. Some people actually choose to fast as a lifestyle, even if they don't have any weight to lose.

Fasting can benefit your entire quality of life in the following ways:

Fasting will help you take the weight off and keep it off.

The reason for the weight loss is pretty straightforward: in eating fewer meals, you're consuming fewer total calories. As long as you don't overcompensate when you're not fasting, fewer calories translates to more pounds lost. As a bonus, hormonal changes as your body adapts to fasting will enhance your metabolic function to burn calories more efficiently and contribute to the weight loss. Some of that weight loss is in the abdominal area, the harmful belly fat that can lead to disease and other health problems. In most cases, you don't even need to count calories.

When you are in the habit of regularly eating three meals a day, and sometimes more, the food is converted to glucose for energy. It takes about 10 to 12 hours for the body to use up a single supply of glucose from one meal. As long as you are providing a constant supply of fuel, there will be no need for the body to turn to its own fat stores to get energy.

In studies comparing obese individuals on an intermittent fasting regimen with others on a traditional diet plan, both groups were able to successfully achieve a lower Body Mass Index (BMI), but the IF group showed a reduced tendency to put weight back on after a period of one year.

Fasting will allow your digestive system to rest, repair, and revitalize.

This seems pretty obvious. If you don't have food coming in all the time, you don't need to digest anything. The digestive organs don't just stand by, though. There are still processes going on in the body to eliminate toxins and waste from the body.

Fasting can allow you to enjoy a longer, more robust lifespan.

It may not be the Fountain of Youth, but there have been some studies that indicate that fasting can actually slow down the aging process, as well as help fight off age-related disease. Apparently, going without food for a more than a normal length of time causes your body to respond at a cellular level to what it perceives as a situation of stress. Once a stressful situation is identified, the cells make adaptations to deal with it. As a result, your body is not only able to cope better with the stress of fewer energy-giving calories, but it also has the ability to deal with other stressors, such as disease. According to an article in the journal *Gerontology*, animal studies have shown that rats that are given alternate day fasting schedules have lived as much as 83% longer than rats on a traditional diet. They have also demonstrated a lower incidence of cancers and age-related disorders such as coronary artery disease, stroke, and Alzheimer's. As more human studies are completed, intermittent fasting could well become the go-to strategy for optimum health and a better life.

Intermittent fasting may help reduce the risk for developing diabetes.

As the incidence of overweight and obesity grows, so does the rate of type 2 diabetes. The number of people diagnosed with prediabetes has reached alarming levels. Prediabetes is a wakeup call to lose weight and start living a healthy lifestyle so that you don't become another diabetes 2 statistic. There are two terms to consider here: insulin sensitivity, which is good, and insulin resistance, which is not good.

When you are insulin-resistant, your pancreas is not producing enough insulin to keep your blood sugar levels under control. When your blood sugar is too high, you may be headed for type 2 diabetes, if you're not already there. Losing weight will increase your insulin sensitivity, helping to keep your blood sugar at an acceptable level.

Intermittent fasting has been shown to lower insulin resistance so that the blood sugar level drops down as much as 3 to 6 percent, and insulin levels decrease by as much as 20 to 31 percent. This is according to an article on sciencedirect.com.

One of the most serious complications of diabetes is kidney damage. A study on rats showed that they were protected from this condition during intermittent fasting, and their risk of hypertension was lowered.

There is more research to be done before we can say for certain that intermittent fasting can provide these benefits to every individual. Some results seem to contradict others. For example, women may not experience the same blood sugar reduction as men. One study showed that a period of 22 days of intermittent fasting actually showed unfavorable blood sugar results in women. This is just more evidence that every type of protocol needs to be adopted with a high degree of caution and an eye for individual responses.

Intermittent fasting may lead to a lower risk of cardiovascular disease.

According to the CDC, heart disease is the leading cause of death for men and women. Lifestyle habits such as smoking, excess alcohol, and sedentary behaviors all contribute to heart disease risk, and changing these habits can affect your risk dramatically. But intermittent fasting is another factor that can help reduce risk. Studies show that many of the benefits of intermittent fasting--lowered blood pressure, blood sugar levels, insulin levels, LDL and total cholesterol, inflammation, and triglycerides--are the very factors that support cardiovascular health.

Intermittent fasting triggers a "reboot" of the hormones and genes in your body.

We know that the process of consuming any type of calories, healthy or unhealthy, sets off a chain of events to digest and assimilate the nutrients. But restricting the calories does not mean that the body is just going to rest and do nothing. The digestive organs may get a rest, but the tiny machines that run your metabolism become very active. When you fast, your pancreas can take a break from producing insulin, but your pituitary gland sends out an extra supply of human growth hormone (HGH). Even though you technically stopped growing once you reached adulthood, HGH is still vital for cell regeneration. When it's produced at higher levels, your body burns more fat while slightly increasing muscle mass.

Fasting also initiates changes in gene expression, the code that tells your cells what their function will be. Some of these changes affect disease prevention and longevity, as discussed earlier. In addition, according to *The Scientist* magazine, a recent study of fasting rats showed that the change in gene expression improved their ability to learn, and their brains were more like those of their younger counterparts.

Intermittent fasting helps in the process of cell repair.

Our bodies have a natural defense against aging or damaged cells: It eats them. This process is called *autophagy*, which derives from the Greek terms for "self" and "eat." It's a way the body has to recycle or eliminate waste matter and allow cells to repair themselves. For obvious reasons, it's a process that must stay under strict control, but when fasting reduces the levels of vital nutrients, including glucose, your body senses a need for more food, and autophagy is initiated. This speeds up the process of clearing the body of broken-down proteins that tend to build up within cells over time. Removing these dysfunctional proteins is believed to protect against diseases such as cancer and Alzheimer's.

Intermittent fasting can lead to a reduction in inflammation and oxidative stress in the body and strengthen your immune system.

Over the past few decades, researchers have become aware of a class of molecules known as free radicals and the harmful effects they have on our bodies when they are out of control. Free radicals are molecules that are unstable and attack other molecules, including DNA, proteins, and enzymes, causing damage. On the plus side, some of this damage produces toxins that our immune systems can use to fight infection. Inflammation is a normal part of these defenses, but it's a sign that the body is trying to heal itself.

However, when there is an overproduction of free radicals, it can create unnecessary and undesirable inflammatory responses, which can lead to a long list of harmful effects such as cancer, heart disease, cerebrovascular disease (stroke), emphysema, rheumatoid arthritis, ulcers, cataracts, dementia, osteoporosis, premature aging of the skin, muscle stiffness, and more.

Our bodies produce free radicals because of a number of internal and external factors. They are a byproduct of the many metabolic functions of our cells. So when we digest food, exercise, experience stress, spend time in the sun, or expose ourselves to environmental pollutants, we produce free radicals. Smokers and drinkers get an extra dose of these potential bad guys.

The instability of free radicals is because they are essentially incomplete molecules; they lack an electron. This is a result of the process of oxidation, the same process that turns an apple brown when it's exposed to oxygen. When free radicals are overproduced, it leads to oxidative stress. Several studies have concluded that intermittent fasting can also boost metabolic defenses against oxidative stress. Our bodies have some natural defense mechanisms against oxidative stress, but sometimes they need a boost by supplying them with antioxidant foods, so it's good to add those to your food plan on non-fasting days.

IF also helps revitalize your immune system by activating stem cells. These are the cells that can technically become any kind of cell that the body is in need of. It also restricts the activity of a gene called PKA. This is the gene that generates an enzyme that inhibits the regeneration of cells, so restricting its activity allows your body to go about its business of repairing cells.

Intermittent fasting has benefits for your brain.

So far, we have shown that intermittent fasting can lead to a reduction of oxidative stress, a lower rate of inflammation, reduced blood sugar levels, and lowered insulin resistance, all very beneficial for the body. But these same results are also important for the development and preservation of a healthy brain. As studies continue, more evidence is discovered that the process of autophagy creates pathways to establish new neurons and build synapses between them.

This process is complemented by BDNF (Brain-Derived Neurotrophic Factor) which is a protein in the brain that impacts function of both the brain and the peripheral nervous system. Fasting initiates an increase in BDNF, which supports existing brain cells while generating the growth of new neurons and synapses. In animal studies, a low level of BDNF is associated with depression, loss of memory, and diminished cognitive ability. For example, one study of BDNF-deficient rats showed that they had more trouble finding their way through a maze than their counterparts in the control group or even remembering where to find food.

While most of the organs have a reduction in size with a restricted calorie diet, animal studies show that the brain's size is not affected. This seems to point to an evolutionary trait that our ancestors developed as a defense against starvation. When food was scarce, they needed to have more brain power to seek out food while avoiding predators, so their brains received nutrients while other organs may have been deprived.

There is also some evidence that intermittent fasting enables the brain to repair itself from injury and disease, including damage from stroke. Moreover, in animal studies of cervical spine injury, rats who were fasting alternate days were able to regain movement and function that depend on proper brain function.

One of the most annoying effects of aging is cognitive decline--loss of memory, difficulty processing information and making decisions, problems with concentration, struggle to communicate, brain fog, etc. But there's hope in the form of IF. An article in *Age (Dordr)*, a journal out of the Netherlands, reported that some research has shown that Intermittent fasting actually halted mental decline in rats, even the older ones who were already showing signs of deterioration.

Another benefit that intermittent fasting has for the brain is in treatment of seizures due to epilepsy. Preliminary research is ongoing, but several studies have shown that children and adults who suffer from epilepsy experienced a lower number of episodes after fasting. Some of them had a reduction by as much as 99 percent when they hadn't had much success with medication.

Intermittent fasting may help prevent Alzheimer's disease.

Even though we've discussed it in other sections, Alzheimer's disease is such a troubling topic that it deserves a section of its own. Alzheimer's, a neurodegenerative disease that starts out slowly and gets progressively worse as the patient gets older, is the main force behind 60 to 70 percent of all cases of dementia. Although people who typically suffer from the disease are seniors who have reached 65 years of age or older, a small percentage of younger people have been known to develop the disease. It's a devastating problem, not just for the person who develops the disease, but also for loved ones who must assume the role of caregiver.

Early symptoms of Alzheimer's are mild, mostly some memory loss, but as the disease progresses, it becomes more and more difficult to function in simple daily activities. A person can live anywhere from four to twenty years with the disease after they demonstrate visible symptoms; the average survival time is eight years. At this point there is no cure, although some treatments have been developed to alleviate the symptoms and slow the deterioration process.

That's why it is vital for people of any age to do anything they can do to prevent its onset. Intermittent fasting is one simple lifestyle change that could accomplish that goal. One article published in the journal *Aging* reported a study of ten patients who were suffering from different levels of cognitive dysfunction. They were placed on a protocol that included intermittent fasting and, after three to six months, there was a significant improvement in nine out of ten patients in the study group. The patient who did not respond successfully was already in late stage Alzheimer's. This is a small study, but the results are unquestionably promising for potential prevention of Alzheimer's.

Intermittent fasting can reduce the risk of some cancers.

Since intermittent fasting works on so many levels of your metabolic system, some of these benefits may add another benefit: avoiding cancer. So far, most research involves animal studies, but the results definitely warrant more investigation via human studies. One particular study reported by Bojan Kostevski, M.D., involved a particular classification of mice that have a tendency to develop lymphoma after a certain age. The fasting mice were fed every other day while a control group was allowed to feed at will. After 16 weeks, 33 percent of the feeding mice developed lymphomas, while none of the fasting mice did.

While this is a good reason for mice to celebrate, we humans should reserve final judgment until human studies have shown similar results, but since we're all mammals, the chances look good. There is some good news for humans, however. Some studies have shown that human cancer patients have experienced reduced side effects from chemotherapy while fasting. Again, more studies must be done to support these findings, but there's every reason to be optimistic about intermittent fasting as a defense against cancer.

Intermittent fasting can boost your spiritual side.

Even when you're a gung ho, all in, totally enthusiastic practitioner of fasting, there is still an element of sacrifice to it. After all, you're giving up one of your standard worldly comforts, even if it is only temporary. As you pay less attention to food and all that goes with it, you naturally redirect your focus internally. In the early stages of fasting there will likely be hunger pangs, but as your body becomes accustomed to the changes you're asking it to make you will find a quiet place within to connect with the universe. You will notice that you feel lighter in body and in spirit. If you choose to meditate or pray, you will be more focused and less distracted by things of the physical world. Your intellect will become sharper, and you will also be more intuitive and insightful. Spirituality is a personal thing, so you may experience a closer relationship with your creator, or you may find a better understanding of your fellow man. In any case, you will feel a deeper consciousness and contentment because you are more able to let go of your worldly burdens.

Intermittent fasting can help build character.

Hopefully, you're not scoffing in disbelief at this idea, because it's actually true. IF can reach into your inner consciousness and pull out positive traits that will make you a better person. The development of self-discipline is obvious; it takes plenty of self-control to ignore the hunger pangs and stay with the program until it's time to break the fast. But many people who fast believe that they have developed greater empathy and compassion. When you think about it, it makes sense. Technically, you are making a sacrifice, and you may be suffering a little bit by making it. This experience can help you better understand the suffering of others.

As more research is conducted on intermittent fasting, more benefits and potential benefits are discovered. But even without the scientific research, there are actual practitioners who swear that some form of intermittent fasting has transformed their lives. Celebrities like Beyoncé and Hugh Jackman and others have followed some form of IF. It has even become a kind of subculture in Silicon Valley where tech execs claim they have lost weight and gained mental clarity and increased focus. Many of them even report feeling "euphoric" while on the fast.

Research into this phenomenon continues, and hopefully science will soon support all the anecdotal evidence of the benefits of intermittent fasting. Until then, there will continue to be mixed messages from the health community and the public.

THE SCIENCE BEHIND INTERMITTENT FASTING

Although fasting of any kind has been around for centuries, it is only recently that scientific research has begun to ask and answer questions about its effects. We are slowly beginning to understand what happens to our bodies when we fast and the effects fasting has on our systems. We've already discussed some of these processes in an earlier section, but now it's time to get into a little more detail.

The first thing your body does when you abstain from taking in any calories is change your hormone levels so that it can continue getting fuel for energy. After about 12 hours of a fast, the glucose you had been getting from food is depleted. As your glucose levels drop, your pancreas doesn't need to produce insulin to keep your blood sugar level under control. Insulin is the hormone that your body uses to process glucose and keep your blood sugar under control. It's an essential component for you to assimilate the food you eat because too much glucose in your system is toxic. When your insulin levels are lower, your store of body fat becomes more readily available.

Once your body is no longer able to find glucose to use as fuel, it has to resort to the glycogen stores in your liver and muscles. Then, when all the glycogen has been consumed, it's time to turn to the fat stores.

At this point the fatty acids produce ketone bodies to provide energy for your brain and body.

Another hormone that kicks into high gear when you fast is HGH, Human Growth Hormone. The levels of this hormone can reach as high as five times their normal levels when you fast. This also helps in using up stored fat, but in addition, it will help prevent muscle loss and may even help you actually gain muscle in some cases. Studies of men over 60 also showed a slight reduction in bone loss and less thinning of the skin.

Norepinephrine, or adrenaline, is another hormone that is affected when you fast. You may be aware of this stress hormone as the "fight or flight" hormone because it kicks in an extra boost of energy when you are faced with danger. One of its other functions is to communicate with your body to break down fat cells into fatty acids. When you fast, you get a boost of norepinephrine in your bloodstream, which means that you have more available fat to burn. As a side benefit, you will have improved focus.

And then there's IGF-1, insulin-like growth factor-1. This is a hormone that supports the active growth of cells. While this seems like it would be a good thing for your body, and it is when you're young and growing, once you get older IGF-1 can actually speed up the aging process, and some studies suggest that there is a connection between high IGF-1 levels and the development of cancers of the prostate, colon, and breasts. Fasting reduces IGF-1 production so that your body can stay younger longer, and you will have a lower risk of cancer. There is also some evidence that indicates that these levels remain lower for a time after you break the fast.

The lower IGF-1 levels applied to groups in a study that compared two groups who ate the same number of calories in a day: one group ate the calories in the traditional 3 meal pattern, while the other group fasted for 16 hours and then ate the calories within an 8 hour window. The group that fasted showed an appreciable difference in the lowering of IGF-1 levels, while the control group saw no difference.

One of the biggest obstacles to controlling hunger during a fast, or any other calorie restricting diet is the hormone ghrelin, also known as the hunger hormone. When you have gone without food for a certain period of time, ghrelin kicks in and tells your brain that you MUST EAT--NOW! This feeling is very strong as ghrelin levels increase in the beginning of a fast, but most people are able to keep the hunger under control by drinking fluids. However, if you absolutely cannot handle the hunger pangs and you feel terrible, there's nothing wrong with admitting that fasting may not be for you.

That's the downside of ghrelin. But there is an upside to having increased levels of ghrelin in your system. If you can overcome the hunger pangs that ghrelin produces, you will be able to reap the rewards of its other effects. Ghrelin facilitates the release of HGH, which we talked about earlier. But it also augments the effects of dopamine, which will work in your brain to give you a feeling of well-being and improve your mood. Ghrelin is also an important factor in maintaining healthy neurons in your brain, specifically the hippocampus, to improve memory and other cognitive function.

Aside from hormonal activity, there are two processes that involve keeping the body's cells healthy and strong: autophagy, which was mentioned earlier, and apoptosis. These are normal processes in the body, but they move rather slowly. Fasting accelerates these processes to different degrees, depending on factors unique to an individual.

Apoptosis is the process that seeks out aging, deteriorating cells that are no longer viable, and may actually lead to conditions like allergies, autoimmune disorders, and in some cases, even conditions like multiple sclerosis. When these cells are identified by markers, the body destroys the entire cell, like demolishing a house, breaking them down into amino acids that the body can use for fuel. This action gets a boost during a longer fast, after about three days or so.

Autophagy, on the other hand, can rev up as early as 12 hours into a fast. This process targets the cells that may be full of toxins, viruses, bacteria, deteriorated proteins, and other trash, and it clears them out. That's more like spring cleaning, leaving the house intact. The longer the duration of the fast, the cleaner the house.

In both of these instances the body burns the undesirable debris for fuel. When you go back to consuming calories, the processes slow back down because your body no longer needs to work so hard to fuel itself.

Depending on what state your body is in as you begin to fast, the time it takes for autophagy to set in can vary. If you have a large supply of glycogen stored in your liver and muscles, it will take longer for the fuel to be consumed so that autophagy can begin. If you resume eating before the glycogen is depleted, autophagy won't initiate at all.

On the other hand, if glycogen stores are relatively low, as they are in people who follow a diet with low carbohydrates, higher fats, and just the right amount of protein, like a ketogenic diet, you may already be burning ketones for fuel, and there won't be very much glycogen, so autophagy will kick in earlier. If you have a diet with a high amount of starches, sugars, and other carbs, you may have to fast for 24 hours before you can benefit from autophagy.

Going into a little more detail on this topic, both your body and your brain will benefit from the ketone activity that is triggered by both fasting and a ketogenic diet. In fact, if the brain had a choice, it would rather use ketones for fuel instead of glucose.

Another scientific aspect to consider in intermittent fasting is the body's natural circadian rhythms. These rhythms are the 24 hour cycle of processes that affect our body's sleeping and waking cycles in response to the cycle of daylight and darkness, as well as the changing temperatures of the seasons. These factors were vital for our Paleolithic ancestors in their search for food, which was more available and easier to hunt during daylight hours and more prevalent during certain seasons.

The nutrition patterns that our ancestors established seem to have carried over to our modern times, and there is a different response to eating during the day and eating at night.

A study conducted in 2013 involved assigning diets of 1400 calories per day to women who were classified as overweight or obese. The women were randomly assigned to two groups that we'll call the Breakfast Bunch and the Dinner Divas. Breakfast or dinner would be the meals where each group would consume the greater portion of the day's 1400 calories.

The results were revealing: the Breakfast Bunch experienced greater weight loss than the Dinner Divas, in spite of the fact that both groups were taking in the same number of calories. Some experts say that one reason for this is the fact that we have more time to burn calories earlier in the day. But circadian rhythms also come into play. Most of our hormone secretion is impacted by our circadian rhythms, and apparently, the body's insulin response, which is a factor in weight gain, is greater in the evening. In the case of the Divas, it was as much as 25 to 50 percent greater.

The results of this study give credence to the theory that a hormone imbalance may be as much as, or more of, a factor in obesity than calorie consumption. This could also point to a link between night shift schedules and weight problems.

PART 2: HOW TO FAST

DIFFERENT INTERMITTENT FASTING METHODS

Fasting is a broad term, even for scientists. It can mean going weeks with nothing but water, eating nothing but soup, or just skipping one meal in a day. There are many options when it comes to intermittent fasting, just as there are many personal preferences. Each of the following methods has its own protocol and varying degrees of benefits. The methods in this section all promise to lead to weight loss and health benefits, but the ultimate difference is how an individual can tolerate the restrictions in each method.

Method one: Time-restricted fasting, or the 16/8 Method

This is the method that Martin Berkhan promotes in his LeanGains program. Time-restricted fasting is most appealing to people who find it difficult or impossible to go 24 hours or more without food.

In this method, a person will generally fast for 16 hours and eat high quality foods the other 8. It can also be modified to 12/12, 20/4, or other combinations. In many cases, simply skipping one meal a day does the trick. Since you have to sleep for six to eight hours a night anyway, that counts as part of the fast, so those hours can be subtracted from the time of active fasting. So instead of fasting for 16 hours, subtract the 8 hours when you're asleep, and you're only really consciously depriving yourself of food for the remaining 8 hours.

Your sixteen-hour fasting time could be from 8:00 PM to noon the next day, or, if you tend to feel hungrier in the morning, you might choose to eat a good breakfast and have your eating period from 7:00AM to 3:00 PM. You don't have to limit the number of meals you eat during the eight hours, but you should make sure that you're eating wholesome food, not junk, and you should try not to overstuff yourself in anticipation of the fasting period. If you have planned a workout during the day, your meals should be a bit higher in healthy carbs (not refined). If it's a low-energy day, your meals should include a little more healthy fats.

During the fasting period, you cannot eat anything, but you should drink plenty of fluids: Mostly water is best, but you can also have black coffee, hot or iced tea, and other no-calorie beverages. Staying hydrated is just good practice, but it also helps to keep those hunger pangs from distracting you too much. It's also important to maintain a consistent schedule of fasting/eating times so that your hormones don't become disrupted.

Method two: The Two Meal Day method

This method, conceived by personal trainer Max Lowery, is very similar to the 16:8 diet, but its main focus is to have a specific number of meals in a day, rather than watching the clock and eating at will during a certain time window. The meals could be breakfast and lunch, or they could be lunch and dinner, but the point of this diet is to set a routine and stick to it. Max is also very involved in fitness training, and he agrees with other experts who recommend keeping carb intake higher on workout days and lower on resting days. Like the Paleo Diet and many others, he also recommends avoiding refined carbohydrates like white bread and pasta and substituting foods like quinoa, brown rice, and sweet potatoes to get your carbs. In addition, Max advocates going meatless for three days and always keeping hydrated by drinking plenty of fluids. The Two Meal Day method doesn't have any restrictions on alcohol, but it should be limited to three or four times a week.

Method three: The Eat-Stop-Eat method

This is a 24-hour fast method that is intended to be carried out once or twice a week. In practice, you would eat dinner on day one, then restrict yourself from having any food until dinnertime on day two. If you wanted to modify it, you could choose to fast between breakfast or lunch instead. Following the fasting period, you would resume normal eating patterns until the next "Stop" day. No need to count calories, carbs, or fats. According to Brad Pilon, who is the developer of this method, you can even indulge in a little treat now and then, within reason, of course; moderation is the only rule during the eating phase of this method.

Eat-Stop-Eat is an effective method of weight loss for the simple fact that by cutting down your hours of eating, you are reducing your overall calories. Even people who tend to break a fast by "pigging out" would have a hard time replacing the calories they missed during a 24 hour fast. This method also calls for including a regular workout schedule with a focus on weight training to ensure muscle integrity.

The Eat-Stop-Eat fasting method is also designed to be flexible so that beginners can ease into it gradually. If 24 hours is overly difficult, you can just fast until you feel you must eat something or you will die (Be sure you're being honest with yourself, though). As your body begins to adjust, and you progress toward more fasting days, you can gradually build up to the 24-hour fasting goal. It does take a lot of self-discipline to get through the entire 24 hours.

Method four: the 5:2 Diet, or Modified Fasting

Some people find this diet easier to stick to because the time for fasting does not completely restrict eating. This is a weekly cycle where you have two non-consecutive days, for example, Monday and Thursday, where you reduce your normal intake of calories to only 25 percent of your usual consumption. This means that women will eat about 500 calories and men will eat about 600. The calories can be consumed in one sitting, or they may be spread out over the day. On the other five days, you can follow a normal diet.

Dr. Michael Mosley treated himself as a guinea pig on this program and experienced significant results in weight loss and health benefits. As a result, he wrote the best-selling book, *The Fast Diet* to inform the public about the 5:2 diet and his personal experience. Dr. Mosley created this diet to be a permanent lifestyle change, but at some point he discovered that his weight loss was continuing after he had reached his desired weight, so he modified his fasting schedule to one day out of six. He says that if he gains a few pounds because of holiday splurging, he returns to the 5:2 protocol to take off the extra weight fast.

Just as with the other plans, whether it's a limited calorie (fasting) day or a normal calorie day, it's important to eat wholesome foods, and only until you feel satisfied. (You may not reach that point on a fasting day, but you can calm your hunger pangs to a degree.) Bingeing or grabbing unhealthy junk food isn't good for anybody, and it may actually reverse any progress that you make.

Although there is no list of approved foods that you can eat on a fasting day--or for that matter, on a feeding day--you should use good judgment and stick to wholesome foods. Eating junk food with empty calories can undermine any health benefits that you get from fasting. There is also no rule about when you should have your small meals. Some people must have something in their stomach to start off the day, so they might have a small breakfast, maybe an egg and a piece of fruit. Others may be perfectly satisfied to wait until later in the day to eat anything.

In addition, some people feel the need to space out the allowed calories over three smaller meals, and others prefer to have a few more calories in two meals. This would be one case of intermittent fasting where you might find it necessary to keep track of calories. For best results, foods with a high protein, as well as high-fiber foods are the best choices for helping you to feel satisfied on fewer calories. Some good choices include eggs, yogurt, vegetables, fish, lean meat, poultry, soups, and berries. To drink, you can include plenty of water, black coffee, black, green, or herbal tea, or other zero-calorie beverages. If you must include diet soda, be sure to keep it to a minimum.

Later on in this book you will find some suggested meal plans that will help you plan.

Method five: Alternate Day Fast, a.k.a. Up Day, Down Day

The Alternate Day Fasting method is just what it sounds like: fasting one day, feeding the next day, repeat, and repeat, and so on. It basically takes the 5:2 method and adds one more fasting day so that it's a 4:3 program. Studies conducted on this method found that participants lost an average of 3 to 8 percent of their body weight within a period of 24 weeks with no decrease in metabolism.

The Up Day Down Day version of the program was developed by James Johnson, M.D., and it's a modified version where you can eat up to one-fifth of your normal calories on a fasting day. That translates to only about 400 to 500 calories.

Method six: The Warrior Diet

Fitness guru Ori Hofmekler developed this diet, which is not a true fast, but the calorie consumption for 20 hours of each day is strictly limited. During those 20 hours, you can eat only raw vegetables and fruit for most of the day, then have a substantial dinner within a four-hour window. The emphasis on this diet is natural, unprocessed whole foods, similar to the Paleo Diet.

This diet isn't necessarily targeted at weight loss, but it is intended to reduce fat and improve fitness levels, as well as provide some of the health benefits mentioned earlier.

As a soldier (warrior) in the Israeli army, Hofmekler noticed that he and his friends functioned better when they did not eat very much during the time they were most active, the daytime, and reserved most of their calorie consumption to the time when the day's activities were finished, and they could take it easy. In his experience, eating the six to seven meals the army provided, plus snacks, actually made him more fatigued, both physically and mentally. When he did some research on the subject, he found that warriors from past armies had followed a pattern of eating less during the day and more in the evening. So the Warrior Diet was born.

The Warrior Diet is basically a daily cycle of under-eating, where the warrior can eat small amounts of raw fruits or vegetables, some protein such as yogurt or fresh juice. This 20-hour under-eating period is followed by a 4 hour window in the evening in which you can eat a substantial meal of wholesome food. You should start off by having vegetables, some protein, and some good fats. If you still feel hungry, you can then add some more carbohydrates.

The main principle of the diet depends more on human instinct than control. Rather than having strict rules to follow regarding calories, fats, or carbohydrates, you listen to your body and eat accordingly. An important component of the undereating phase includes an exercise regimen that

Hofmekler calls Controlled Fatigue Training (CFT). This means that exercise occurs during the time that you are calorie deprived and may already be feeling fatigue. Hofmekler maintains that this type of exercise activates the genes we have inherited from our caveman ancestors, who had to hunt, run, or fight when their energy levels were not at their highest level.

This method carries a bit more controversy with it than some of the other methods, but there are many practitioners who claim that it is just the right program for them.

Method seven: Fat Loss Forever

In the Fat Loss Forever plan, John Romaniello and Dan Go wrote the book, literally. In fact, they published their program in ten volumes called--what else?--*Fat Loss Forever*. Roman, as Romaniello prefers to be called, is a fitness expert and author, and Dan, also a fitness expert, is well-known internationally as a fitness boot camp instructor.

Together, they conceived the notion of combining all the best factors of Warrior Diet, Eat-Stop-Eat, and Leangains into one unified program, and then threw in a cheat day. The cheat day is an incentive to get ready for the 36 hour fast that follows, and then the next three days each have different fasting procedures. The result is a 12 week program of nutrition and exercise that aims at helping to burn fat faster than traditional diets and keep you at your ideal weight and health level for the rest of your life.

This program requires more attention to detail than some of the others since each day of the week has a different protocol. This type of regimented structure helps some people to stay focused and on track. On the other hand, others may find the schedule a bit confusing. The program has that covered, though, with the inclusion of a planning calendar that specifies the exercise and eating patterns for each day.

Method eight: The Crescendo Method

This method was developed in recognition of the fact that some women, especially women of reproductive age, experience hormonal and fertility problems with intermittent fasting. This method allows women to gradually ease into the practice of fasting so that they avoid any hormone disruption. You never fast on consecutive days on this program, and the fasting window is 12-16 hours.

For some people, following a prescribed program is too much of a burden, and they find their own ways to practice intermittent fasting. They feel that they are already in tune with their bodies, so they may just randomly skip a meal or two every now and then. Some people even go for a day or two every few weeks without eating. This illustrates how intermittent fasting is a very personal mission.

One important thing to remember is this: Although fasting reduces appetite for most people, this is not a permanent change. If you stop fasting for more than a few days, your appetite will return, and you'll be back where you started.

FASTING FOR GENERAL HEALTH

Although fasting has been around for centuries, it has only recently become very popular among the modern masses, and one reason for this is its reputed and proven effects on overall health. We've touched on how fasting helps with epileptic seizures, and many studies are being conducted to discover whether there is an effect on people with multiple sclerosis. But intermittent fasting also seems to help a wide array of general health problems.

Before you get the wrong idea, this is not a "cure" for these ailments; intermittent fasting is a tool to greater health. It merely provides the digestive system an opportunity to rest from the task of dealing with the almost constant assault of food, healthy or unhealthy, that needs to be digested and assimilated. This is a huge job for our body; it's estimated that our digestive organs require as much as 65 percent of the body's energy resources just to process a heavy meal. Without that kind of demand, the body has a chance to recalibrate and switch on "the physician within" (words of Paracelsus, Swiss scientist from the Middle Ages) so that it can begin to heal itself.

As you fast, your body experiences distinct transformations. At first, there may be uncomfortable side effects such as weakness, fatigue, lightheadedness, and headaches. But these should disappear once your body becomes accustomed to the new routine. Then the magic begins to happen: aches and pains may disappear, energy levels begin to soar, skin issues will improve, and you'll just feel better.

But "healing" doesn't stop there. As you make intermittent fasting a lifestyle practice, you may see improvement in so many areas, significant and minor. In some cases, the conditions may actually disappear. But don't expect miraculous results after you practice the 8:16 method for five days and then go back to your old habits. It takes consistency over the long haul to reap the benefits, and sometimes, depending on the condition, it requires a fast of longer duration to achieve the best outcome.

The list below illustrates many of the conditions that can benefit to one degree or another from intermittent fasting. As you can see, there is encouragement and hope for just about any human ailment, physical or mental:

- *Digestive disorders:* ulcerative colitis, irritable bowel syndrome, Crohn's disease, inflammatory bowel disease
- *Cardiopulmonary disorders:* atherosclerosis, high blood pressure, heart disease, high cholesterol
- *Musculoskeletal disorders:* arthritis, joint pain, rheumatoid arthritis, bone density loss, osteoporosis

- *Skin disorders:* acne, eczema, psoriasis, wrinkles
- *Psychological and nervous system disorders:* anxiety, tension, depression, addiction and substance abuse, hyperactivity, chronic fatigue, headaches, insomnia
- *Respiratory disorders:* asthma, hay fever, sinusitis
- *Hormonal disorders*: diabetes, PMS, uterine fibroids, autoimmune disease, hypoglycemia

If help with all of these disorders isn't enough, intermittent fasting also strengthens the immune system with the result that it may lower your chances of catching a cold, the flu, or other infections. In many fasting studies, mostly involving animals at this point, there have even been some forms of cancer that have shown a significant decrease. Of course, it bears repeating that everyone is different, and none of these improvements is guaranteed for every individual. But most people who fast will find that they benefit from a general improvement in health.

FASTING FOR WEIGHT LOSS

Although most fans of intermittent fasting have all kinds of praise for intermittent fasting and the way it makes them feel, there is one benefit that seems to be mentioned more than anything else and that is how easy and fast it is to lose weight when on any of the methods. There are always some, though, who will say it didn't work or it made them feel miserable. They'll show up here and there on a blog or a review and say that intermittent fasting was the biggest mistake they ever made. It's good to get their input; it's a good illustration of just how personal every situation is. (It's also possible that these people didn't do something right.) But these critics are in a minority.

The modern definition of being overweight is having a Body Mass Index (BMI) of 25 to 29. This number is used in determining whether a person has metabolic syndrome, a hodgepodge of symptoms that indicate less than ideal health. If your BMI hits 30 or higher, you're considered obese. Anyone whose BMI is lower than 18.5 is considered underweight, and fasting is probably not a good idea. You need two numbers to determine your BMI: your weight in pounds, and your height in inches. Then you multiply your pounds by 703 and you find your inches squared. Then you divide pounds by inches, and the result is your BMI. If math has never been your strong suit, you can also find BMI calculators online.

Although intermittent fasting is not a goofproof way to lose weight and keep it off, it is a great tool for pointing you in the right direction. It's really up to you how well the tool will work. If you don't have the commitment to really change your behavior and your lifestyle, you will not see the results you're looking for. The good news is that sticking to a fasting protocol actually helps you pay attention to all the aspects of your life, including your weight and your eating habits. You'll get a new perspective, empowering you to realign your focus and broaden your outlook so that making the right choices becomes second nature.

If you carry too much fat around with you, your body is telling you that, even if you're only eating healthy food, you're eating too many calories. Intermittent fasting helps you to cut down on calories overall, as long as you don't overcompensate during the periods you're allowed to eat. Studies have shown that people on some type of intermittent fasting regimen have reduced their weight anywhere from 3 to 8 percent over a 3 to 24 week period. That amounted to anywhere from one to slightly over one-and-a-half pounds per week. There was evidence that the loss included belly fat because their waist measurements went down four to seven percent.

You may hear stories of people who lost amazing amounts of weight instantly, like four pounds in a day, every day, but these stories, while inspiring, can't be true. While some people may experience more impressive weight loss than others, the more gradual, steady losses are more typical. Even if they are on an extended fast, they have to eat sometime, and some of the weight is bound to come back.

As with most diets, fasting weight loss is faster and more dramatic in the first stages, but it levels off pretty quickly. You may lose nothing for a day or two, and some days you might even gain a pound or two. People who carry larger amounts of excess weight will see faster progress. There's also the question of metabolism. If your metabolism is slow, the weight will come off slowly, but it will come off.

Regaining some weight when the fast is over is due to some water weight that occurs when we increase our salt consumption as we go back to eating regular food. This can be a disappointment if you're keeping your eye on the scale all the time. Some people who don't understand how natural this is will even get frustrated and give up and go back to overeating. It's a good idea to restrict scale-watching to once a week, but even then, don't allow a slowdown to discourage you.

Over the long haul, simply engaging in the practice of fasting to lose weight creates more of an awareness of your body's response to real hunger or imagined hunger. Making the right decisions about food will become more organic and won't be influenced by external factors like sights, smells, and advertising. As you begin to understand your eating habits, you will be better able to control them, and you can make the lifestyle changes that will keep you at your ideal weight for a lifetime. Then, if you want to continue to enjoy the other benefits of fasting, you can continue as needed.

FASTING FOR MUSCLE GAIN

People, especially men, who are interested in building muscle are often skeptical about intermittent fasting, holding on to the belief that they will lose muscle along with fat. It's true that an extended fast will ultimately lead to the breakdown of muscle tissue, but if you keep your fasting period short, as in the 16:8 diet, you will still be able to benefit from muscle gain, as long as you follow a few other basic requirements.

The formula for gaining muscle starts out basically in the same way as the formula for gaining fat. If you take in more calories than you burn, your body will convert them to both fat and lean protein mass, which is muscle. But for the best muscle gain, your calorie consumption should include enough protein for muscle building, and you must include an exercise regimen that includes weight training.

In the grand scheme of things, fasting is probably not the most effective way to gain muscle mass. Historically, most weight loss plans result in muscle loss as well as fat loss. But some research does show that resistance training can limit or prevent the loss of muscle. The research in this area is limited because more interest has been focused on the other benefits of fasting, particularly weight loss. Even so, there are a few studies, some which actually focus on the benefits of exercise with intermittent fasting.

One such study involved a group of 34 young men who were divided into two groups. One group followed a normal diet, while the other group was placed on a 16:8 intermittent fasting plan. The number of calories and the amount of protein for both groups were the same, and both groups engaged in the same amount and type of weight training three times a week. The only difference was the scheduling of the eating window. At the end of the 16 week study period, the fasting group had taken off 3.5 pounds of fat, but both groups had maintained their strength and muscle mass. Other health markers in the fasting group also showed improvement.

Similarly, a study involving obese subjects explored the effects of alternate day fasting when combined with endurance exercise. The subjects were randomly divided into four groups: The control group ate a normal diet and followed their normal life style, the second group followed an alternate day fast, the third group ate normally but followed an exercise regimen of 25-40 minutes on an elliptical or stationary bicycle three times a week, and the fourth group followed an alternate day fast with the same exercise regimen. With the exception of the control group, all the other groups were able to lose fat, and had a reduction in waist measurement, but only the fasting/exercise group maintained muscle mass.

The results of both of these studies, and others, is clear: To maintain muscle mass during intermittent fasting, it's essential to include some form of exercise. But it's also important to make sure you're getting enough protein, preferably high-quality animal protein. The recommended amount is about .8 grams of protein, more or less, per pound of body weight when you are trying to maintain muscle. If you want to build muscle, it may be necessary to increase the amount of protein you consume. If you're also trying to lose weight, it's important to be patient and keep the rate of weight loss slow. There's a greater chance of losing muscle mass when the pounds are coming off too rapidly. Try to keep it down to no more than one or two pounds lost per week.

Gaining muscle while on an intermittent fast requires some attention on your part. You need to make sure of three factors:

1) You are getting sufficient exercise to stress the muscles so that the muscle fibers become "damaged." This will initiate the repair process to rebuild them. Autophagy is an essential dynamic in this process. The repaired tissue reinforces the muscle fibers so that your muscles become denser and stronger.
2) You are getting enough calories for basic daily function plus cell repair for your new muscle tissue.

3) You are taking in enough protein to synthesize and replace the protein you are breaking down.

As a rule, intermittent fasting doesn't require you to keep track of the calories you consume, but you may want to modify that rule when it comes to gaining muscle. If you can't maintain a sufficient intake of calories, gaining muscle will be a long, slow process. But it's just as important to make sure you are getting those calories from high quality proteins, carbohydrates, and fats.

There are some people who claim that intermittent fasting is not the best way to gain muscle. Possibly they have had a bad personal experience with it, or perhaps they don't have all the proper information. This is another area where only you, and possibly your doctor, can make the final decision about whether this approach to muscle gain is right for you.

INTERMITTENT FASTING FOR WOMEN

So far, we've discussed many aspects of intermittent fasting, but we need to address the issues of a particular group of people: women. Now we know that fasting causes the body to undergo many changes, and for the most part, they are beneficial for most people. But for women, some of the hormonal changes can potentially lead to an imbalance, and there is a possibility of problems with fertility.

When a woman gets that feeling that she's going to die if she doesn't get something to eat, it's not imaginary or psychological, it's hormonal. The problem lies in women's heightened sensitivity to the hunger hormones, leptin, insulin, and ghrelin. When women go without food for longer than normal, the ghrelin kicks in with a vengeance, and the body believes it's starving; for women, this is all about an inherent need to survive, another attribute that goes back to the times when food was not easily obtained-- genes again. Our ancestors were programmed to survive, not just as individuals, but as a species. For women, this survival concern included potential offspring.

Evidence that intermittent fasting could cause reproductive problems was discovered in a study of female rats who were on intermittent fasting protocols. After just two weeks, the female rats experienced more adverse effects than the males who were on the same protocol. Their menstrual cycles were interrupted, their ovaries began to shrink, and they were unable to reproduce. They also experienced more significant insomnia than the males. Scientists think that the reason for the sleeplessness was a ferocious need to think, plan, and find food.

Unfortunately, although there is an abundance of intermittent fasting studies on human males, there is a shortage of studies of females and even fewer studies on the differences and similarities between fasting males and females. But the animal studies have provided enough information for researchers to reach the conclusion that intermittent fasting can potentially upset hormonal balance for women, possibly even stopping ovulation, and create reproductive problems.

In the few human studies on fasting men and women that have been conducted, there have been some areas where women's responses differed significantly from the men's: The women did not achieve the increase in insulin sensitivity, and their glucose tolerance actually decreased. These differences had detrimental effects on women's metabolisms, and many of them reported undesirable side effects such as anxiety, irritability, insomnia, skin problems, and menstrual irregularity.

On the other hand, there have been some women who report feeling great while following an IF protocol. Reasons for these disparities are not clear; this further illustrates the need for more research studies. In any case, women should approach intermittent fasting with caution. Take it slow and be alert for any negative consequences. If any side effects become evident, it's time to give up on the idea of intermittent fasting. Additionally, there will probably be some days when those hormones become so overpowering that you can't ignore them. Those days are not good days for fasting, so have something to eat, and try again the next day.

Finally, any woman who is already having fertility issues should not think about IF. Similarly, if she is pregnant, trying to get pregnant, or breastfeeding, intermittent fasting should definitely *not* be part of her life.

PART 3: NUTRITION

COMMON MISTAKES WHEN INTERMITTENT FASTING

When you first start out on an intermittent fasting program, the prospects of reaping the benefits can be very exciting. As you look forward to meeting the slimmer, healthier, clearer-thinking new person that will be you, you may lose a bit of focus and make some mistakes along the way. Many people have already made those mistakes, so this list is to help you avoid repeating them so that your progress will be smooth and free of obstacles and setbacks.

- Mistake number one: Convincing yourself that "just a little something to eat" during the fasting phase will not hurt your progress. The truth is that the magic of fasting is centered around the process of autophagy, and a snack or a small meal can disrupt that process. There are different schools of thought on this. Some claim that you should not even add milk or cream to your coffee or tea during the fasting period, while there are others who believe that an indulgence that falls under 50 calories (for the whole period) is harmless. The bottom line seems to be that you can try a little extra if you're desperate, but if you don't see any

73

progress, you should stick with completely abstaining from any kind of calories during the fasting period.

- *Mistake number two: Choosing a method that doesn't suit your schedule, lifestyle, or physiological requirements.* Intermittent fasting is not a one-size-fits-all lifestyle change. There are so many different protocols for the sole reason that different people have different biological responses to periods of not eating. Some people would never be able to manage the 5:2 protocol simply because they can't get past the hunger and the side effects of 24 hours with no food. Schedules are also important. You may be in a fasting state, but you have to feed your family. Or you have to entertain clients. Or your friends want to go out on the town. All of these things potentially interfere with a fast. So you have to make a clear analysis of your schedule, your lifestyle, and your biology when you choose a method. The 16:8 method works for many people because they can choose to skip breakfast or dinner, and the time without eating seems to be more manageable than trying to go a whole day or more. It also seems to be easier to work in some of these other things that are part of life with this method. If you do the research, you can probably determine the method that will give you the greatest chance at success.

- *Mistake number three: Overeating between fasting periods.* One of the most attractive components of intermittent fasting is the promise that you can eat whatever you like until you feel full, and you don't have to count calories. Some people incorrectly interpret this as permission to splurge on rich foods and binge on calories. Or they "graze" mindlessly throughout the non-fasting window and have no real idea of how much food they're putting into their body. These practices are absolutely not going to help anyone lose weight or get healthy. Eating "until you feel full" is not the same thing as stuffing yourself with food that you know is not good for you. Sometimes the signal that you're full takes a while to make it to the brain, so it's important to eat slowly. It's also important to keep your calories mostly health-oriented macronutrients: proteins, healthy carbs (i.e. vegetables), and good fats. This is what it will take to keep you feeling satisfied, with plenty of energy, no muscle loss, and a healthy brain. And don't forget to take in enough fiber; that will help get that full feeling, as well as keeping you regular. That's not to say you can't treat yourself to some pizza or a brownie once in a while. You just can't make it your standard operating procedure.

- *Mistake number four: Eating too little.* One reason that overindulgence occurs in mistake number three is that people *aren't* getting enough calories to support their metabolisms. They become so obsessive about losing weight that they think leaving out as many calories as possible will make everything go faster. But this ambitious plan eventually backfires, and fatigue and weakness set in because there isn't enough fuel. Moreover, the starvation hormone ghrelin kicks in in a big way, and your body starts screaming, "FEED ME!" sort of like that carnivorous plant in *Little Shop of Horrors.* (If you haven't seen it, you should check out the movie. Very entertaining, and it might even help curb your appetite.) As a result, many people get to the point that they go way overboard after the fast, they may skip a fasting period, or they may even quit the program. When you want to lose weight, don't be unrealistic about how you get there. Be practical, and don't let your calorie count drop lower than 1200 on a non-fasting day.

- *Mistake number five: Making a full-force frontal attack from the get-go.* It's hard to overrate enthusiasm, but in the case of fasting, you don't want to do too much too soon, or you will undoubtedly get discouraged by the uncomfortable side-effects that can occur in the beginning. Whichever method you choose to adopt, it's better for your body and your psyche to take a kinder, gentler approach to intermittent fasting. You start by just skipping one meal, or you could aim for just a 12 hour fast. When hunger pangs start to be noticeable, a glass of tea, a cup of coffee, or some ice water should keep them at bay for a little while. If the hunger becomes unbearable before you've reached your goal, don't stress your body, but go ahead and have something to eat. You can aim for a longer fast next time, and it should be easier. Add about 30 minutes to the fast each time until you are fasting for the predetermined amount of time. If your regimen includes exercise, you don't want to go whole hog when you're a novice at fasting. As your body gets more accustomed to the rhythms of fasting, you might feel better exercising on a fast, but when you're just starting out, you will probably be better off if you exercise about two hours after you eat. At first, workouts should be on the mild side, or you should skip them altogether. You can step up the intensity level as your body adjusts to the new routine.

- *Mistake number six: Skimping on fluids.* Staying hydrated is important under normal circumstances, but it's even more important when you're not getting your regular calorie load. We get some water from food, so the fact that we're not eating creates a fluid deficit. The effects will be noticeable; you'll have low energy, and you'll most likely suffer from headaches. The hunger pangs will also be harder to control, and you will have a greater chance of falling off the fast wagon.

- *Mistake number seven: Making poor food choices for non-fasting window.* Even with all its benefits, intermittent fasting is not a guarantee of good health. It's important that you get essential nutrients when you are in your non-fasting period. That means that you should choose fresh, wholesome, whole foods--organic when possible--and avoid empty calories and refined and processed foods that can be harmful to your health.

- *Mistake number eight: Fasting too frequently.* Sometimes people get caught up in an idea and take it too far. Intermittent fasting is not intended to be a marathon, and fasting for too many days in a week can work against you. Ideally, a fast should occur on two days a week, and up to four if you're a veteran at fasting. Any more and your body will think it is being starved and go into defense mode. The result will be something like metabolic chaos. In order to determine the best schedule for you, it may take a little trial and error to see at what point your body begins to be uncomfortable. If you reach that point, you should take your fasting back a notch.

INTERMITTENT FASTING AND FLUIDS

About 55 to 70 percent of the human body is made up of water. The brain alone is nearly 70 percent, and the lungs are almost 90 percent. So staying hydrated is always important for a healthy body, no matter what kind of meal plan you are on. Your body needs water for efficient digestion, to keep body temperature level, carry nutrients to cells and transport waste and toxins from the body, and to keep joints lubricated. It's essential for bladder and kidney function, and it impacts energy levels and hunger signals. All that being said, getting through a fasting period is just easier if you maintain a sufficient intake of water.

You need an ongoing supply of water under normal circumstances, but you need to step it up when you work out, when the temperature is hot, and when you fast. The reason fasting calls for more water is that limiting food also limits water. Just about all foods contain some amount of water. Fruits and vegetables are especially good sources of water in food. For example, strawberries, watermelon, lettuce and cucumbers are more than 90 percent water, with other vegetables also having significant amounts of H_2O. There is even water content in meat, poultry, and fish. So if fasting causes you to cut down on the amount of food you eat, you are missing part of the water you need.

Many people, and some experts, believe that drinking water when you're thirsty is a good way to manage your fluid intake, but the truth is that thirst is actually the first sign of dehydration. If you don't drink any fluids when you are feeling thirsty, the symptoms of dehydration intensify:

- Your urine output decreases, and it intensifies in color.
- Your mouth will be dry and cottony feeling.
- You will stop perspiring.
- You will not be able to produce tears.
- You may experience nausea with or without vomiting.
- You will experience muscle cramps.
- You will experience palpitations of the heart.
- You will experience lightheadedness and headaches.
- You will experience confusion and weakness.
- In final stages, dehydration can lead to organ failure, coma, and death.

This list illustrates just how vital fluids are to our wellbeing, and its importance must not be overlooked both when you are in a fasting state and a non-fasting state. During the fasting state, water is best, and you can have sparkling water if you'd like to liven it up a little. But black coffee and tea, as well as green and herbal teas, are also recommended. There are differing opinions on whether you may add milk or cream to these beverages, so that's basically a judgment call on your part. You also have the option of including some other non-caloric beverages, but it's best to keep those to a minimum and rely on pure, unadulterated water.

There is some concern that fasting leads to loss of electrolytes and minerals, but you can compensate for this by adding a pinch of sea salt to your water when you're fasting. When you're not fasting, you can help regain electrolytes and minerals by including mineral-rich green smoothies and bone broth in your food choices. You may also choose to add some vitamin/mineral supplements to your regimen.

FOODS YOU SHOULD EAT

When you think of fasting, you obviously think of a period without food. But every fast, no matter the length of it, eventually is broken. That's when you need to think about what kinds of food you're going to put into your body. As mentioned earlier, you don't want to gravitate to the junk food and treats that you missed. Instead, you need to focus on wholesome, nutritious macronutrients--lean proteins, high-quality, unrefined carbohydrates, and good fats. Balancing your diet with healthy foods will help curb hunger and cravings so that you're not tempted to overeat.

Start with the protein

Protein is the most important part of your diet, whether you want to lose weight or not. Eating protein helps in achieving satiety (that full feeling) and keeping your appetite under control so that you can better manage your calorie consumption. On the other hand, protein also gives your metabolism a boost and enhances your body's ability to burn calories. Together, these two features provide a one-two punch that will help take weight off faster.

Protein is also a fundamental factor in preventing the muscle loss that often occurs with most types of restrictive diets. You want to lose fat, not lean mass, so when you're not fasting you should pay particular attention to how much protein you're getting. Many health/weight loss experts highly recommend that 30 percent of your calories are from protein. That, along with an exercise regimen, will help you hold on to muscle mass, and possibly even make some gains in that area.

The highest quality protein has the full range of necessary amino acids and is found in animal products; feel free to eat anything from the meat, poultry, fish, and dairy categories. Even some lean red meat like steak is not taboo, as long as you're not overdoing. In the fish category, fatty fish such as salmon and herring are especially good because of their high omega-3 fatty acid content. Dairy products such as eggs, milk, yogurt, and cheese are also great sources, and you can include those on your non-fasting days, as long as you're able to tolerate lactose.

Plant products also provide protein, but they don't provide all the amino acids. Beans, especially soy beans, and lentils are good sources of plant protein. Seeds, nuts, and nut butters are also good. Other good plant sources include oats, quinoa, chia seeds, buckwheat, and spirulina. Tofu and hummus are made from soybeans and chickpeas, respectively, so they are also good sources of protein.

Then there are commercially manufactured protein powders, bars, and shakes. These products are good in a pinch, but for the most part it's much better to get your protein from natural, whole food sources. People who are bodybuilders or elite athletes often augment their protein intake with protein supplements, but it's not necessary for the mainstream.

Add healthy carbohydrates for vitamins, antioxidants, and fiber

With all the buzz these days about low carb lifestyle, it's unusual to see an actual recommendation for eating carbohydrates. We're not talking about white bread and pasta here, but a healthy diet depends on balance, and part of that balance includes complex carbohydrates such as fresh fruits and vegetables. Many experts believe that it takes about 150 grams of carbohydrates in a day to ensure that the body functions at full capacity. If carbohydrates are greatly restricted, as they are in many of the popular low carb diets, you can experience several undesirable side effects after just a couple of days. Some of these side effects include skin rashes, diarrhea or constipation, cramping muscles, fatigue, low energy levels, weakness, and a general unwell feeling. Low carb consumption also causes ketosis, which gives a person bad breath, gas, and leads to breakdown of protein and muscle tissue. There is also a loss of water and sodium, and potential dehydration. There are people who advocate the low carb lifestyle that claim to function very well with ketosis, and they say that it has more benefits than drawbacks. Apparently, their bodies are better suited for that type of diet, and that just illustrates that some things work for some people and not so well for others.

Including fruits and vegetables in your food plan means that you not only avoid the undesirable side effects, but you benefit from all the natural vitamins, minerals, and fiber found in them. Sure, you could take a supplement or two, but nothing beats the nutrients that come directly from nature. Fruits, vegetables, and whole grains are also good sources of fiber, so you need them to keep your digestive system moving efficiently, so to speak. Men should have 28-34 grams of fiber every day, and women should have 22- 28 grams.

Good Fats

After decades on the bad foods list, fats--unsaturated fats in particular--have finally earned their place in the formula for a healthy diet. Even saturated fats, mostly found in meat, have become more respectable, as long as they're consumed in moderation. Nowadays, the only fat that is still considered totally evil is transfat, which is man-made for the most part, not natural like the monounsaturated and polyunsaturated fats that are considered the good fats.

You can recognize transfats on food labels as "partially hydrogenated oil"; many times it will actually identify them as transfats. As much as possible, you should avoid any food with these words on the label. Transfats are the bad guys; they raise bad cholesterol and lower good cholesterol, which increases your chances of developing heart disease or stroke. They also have a connection to a higher risk of type 2 diabetes.

Monounsaturated and polyunsaturated fats, on the other hand, are the good guys. These fats actually provide important nutrients that we need and are important because they help reduce LDL cholesterol (the bad cholesterol), and there is evidence from research studies that they have a positive effect on blood sugar and insulin levels.

Monounsaturated fats are a few degrees more useful than polyunsaturated fats; they have anti-inflammatory properties and can decrease the risk of cardiac disease. Olive oil, avocados, and nuts are all good sources of monounsaturated fats. But polyunsaturated fats are also beneficial in many ways. Found in fish, fish oil, algae, seeds, nuts, and leafy green vegetables, these fats are a good source of omega-3 fatty acids, which are essential for brains, cells, and heart.

Polyunsaturated fats also contain omega-6 fatty acids, which work with omega-3 to reduce LDL cholesterol. But consuming too much omega-6 is not a good idea because a higher proportion of omega-6 in relation to omega-3 plays a role in weight gain, inflammation, and some other health issues.

Having the proper balance of omega-3 and omega-6 fatty acids is necessary for many reasons. Among the benefits are:

- Support for heart
- Pancreas health
- Balancing mood and reducing depression symptoms
- Protection from dementia and memory loss
- Help with skin disorders
- Reducing the risk of diseases like heart disease, cancer, and stroke
- Preventing or reducing symptoms of ADHD and bipolar disorder
- Helping to ensure a healthy pregnancy
- Lessening pain from arthritis
- Memory improvement
- Prevention of fatigue

Unfortunately, it's too easy to get more omega-6 than is good for us because it's so prevalent in the food we eat, especially corn and vegetable oils. If the balance gets skewed so that the proportion of omega-6 is much greater than omega-3, it can lead to trouble with blood pressure, water retention, and blood clots that can lead to heart attack or stroke. For this reason, it's important to monitor your unsaturated fats so that you are getting the balance that will do more good than harm.

Saturated fat is a whole other animal, and the jury is still out on this one. Research goes back and forth on whether or not it's good or bad for you, but there is evidence that we need some saturated fat in our diet for immune support, liver function, developing and protecting our cells, and several other necessary operations. The key thing to remember about saturated fat is to keep it reasonable. Going overboard could lend support to the claims that saturated fats cause heart problems.

Fat is the third of the essential macronutrients for keeping you healthy on an intermittent fasting program. A healthy diet can include as much as 30 percent of our calories from fat, according to many experts. Lowering fat consumption, however, doesn't seem to have significant harmful effects. It's not hard to get enough fat; it's in meat, butter, cheese, milk, nuts, oils, and some vegetables, as well as most dessert products. Just make sure that the majority of the fat you're consuming is on the healthy fat list.

Besides the macronutrients, your non-fasting days can include a variety of condiments to make sure what you eat has maximum flavor. Feel free to use salt (unless you're on a sodium-restricted diet), pepper, herbs, and spices to spice up your food. You can even enjoy an occasional dessert, as long as you keep in mind that the calories and sugar will likely slow down your weight loss progress. It's probably best to indulge in desserts only on special occasions. When you're not fasting, you can enjoy most of your favorite beverages, including wine, beer, and spirits. Again, you don't want to go too far with this because overdoing it one evening can mean a lot of difficulty getting back into the fasting routine the next day.

INTERMITTENT FASTING AND THE KETO DIET

Many people are already fans of the ketogenic diet, and they wonder if adding an intermittent fasting regimen will work well with their routine. The answer is yes. Keto dieting involves high amounts of fat, some protein, and very low amounts of carbohydrates, so that the body enters the state of ketosis. This type of diet provides benefits for a lot of people, but adding intermittent fasting to the regimen can accelerate the process of autophagy, which will enhance these benefits.

One of the primary goals of the keto diet is to get into ketosis so that the body is burning fat instead of glucose, thereby producing ketone bodies. When you add intermittent fasting to the mix, you can get into ketosis much faster because the you are not only reducing the amount of carbs you eat but protein and other macros as well.

The reverse is also true; a keto diet enhances intermittent fasting because a keto diet is a kind of carbohydrate "fast" on its own; therefore, when you enter your window of fasting, you already have a leg up. In addition, fasting is actually easier when you've been on a keto diet because the absence of carbohydrates and the satisfying qualities of higher fats help you overcome hunger and cravings, so you don't feel the need to eat.

When you combine the keto diet with intermittent fasting, you intensify the benefits of autophagy. You already know that this is the process where your body cleans out wastes and toxins from your cells. Since both diets have a role in inducing autophagy, the process becomes more efficient, providing even greater benefits and protection against type 2 diabetes and cardiovascular disease. You will also accelerate your weight loss.

The ketogenic diet is of extra benefit in intermittent fasting because it helps to keep your blood sugar stable. While it tends to level out during a fasting period, if you go back to eating carbohydrates in your non-fasting window, you will start to produce glucose again, and your body will go back to using this for energy instead of ketones. As a result, you may get spikes in your blood sugar, which can result in low energy, fatigue, brain fog, etc. On a keto diet, you don't have those blood spikes because you're keeping your carbs to a minimum so that your body continues to rely on ketones for energy and your blood sugar stays level. This also helps you avoid some of the uncomfortable side effects of ketosis, like the "keto flu."

As you know, there is more than one way to do intermittent fasting, and the same rule of thumb applies to keto dieters in choosing which one is right for you. Ideally, you will get results by fasting anywhere between 12 and 48 hours at a time. There are some experts who recommend fasting for three days about three times a year, but that sort of plan is not for everyone. You can "try on" different fasting methods and see how you feel on them. If you feel that you can't manage the hunger, or you have issues with cognitive function or sleep, that method is probably not a good fit for you.

You also need to make sure that you eat the right amount of calories during your eating window. Not enough calories will cause you to be miserable and may create metabolic issues, while too many calories will erase any progress you have made. You can find apps on the Internet to help you calculate how many calories and ketogenic macronutrients you need for your body type and activity level. Use this as a guideline of how you should eat when you're not fasting. You can use a urine strip to keep track of your ketones so that you don't fall out of ketosis from failing to maintain a ketogenic balance.

While intermittent fasting alone is almost completely nonrestrictive regarding what you can eat during your non-fasting windows, combining it with a keto diet comes with a few restrictions. Although you can eat fattier cuts of meat and other fatty things, you must avoid or limit a pretty long list of high carb foods when you're also on a keto diet:

- Anything containing sugar: soda, candy, pastries, fruit juice, etc.
- Grains and grain-based products: bread, cereal, pasta, rice, etc.

- Potatoes, sweet potatoes, carrots, and other starchy root vegetables
- Most fruit: some berries are allowed
- Beans and legumes
- Alcohol
- Unhealthy fat: corn oil and other processed vegetable oils, mayo, etc.
- Most diet products, check labels for sugar and carb content

When you go shopping for what you can eat, you need to be a carb detective. Check labels on diet products, condiments, and sauces to see if there are hidden sugars, carbs, or unhealthy fats. Also check for sugar alcohols in "sugar free" foods. Being unaware of any of these things can affect your ketone levels.

The ketone diet is not for everyone, and intermittent fasting is not for everyone. But they are for many people, who swear that the combination of keto dieting and intermittent fasting is the best thing they've ever done for losing weight and gaining better health and confidence.

SAMPLE MEAL PLANS

Since there are a variety of different styles of fasting methods, this section includes a hodgepodge of meal plans that should address one or more of these methods. The first group of meal plans is for the eating window on the 5:2 plan, where you limit calorie consumption to 500-600 for the day.

5:2 Non-fasting day meal plan

Finding the best way to spread out the 500 to 600 calories you're allowed to eat on a fasting day is probably the trickiest part of the 5:2 diet, and it may take some hits and misses before you come up with the routine that works best for you. Many people claim to have good luck by spreading the calories out over four to five meals during the day, but that makes the meals very small. Others are comfortable eating their calories in just two sittings. As much as possible, each meal should include fresh vegetables and fruits. The meal plans offered here are basically suggestions about what you can realistically eat on the 5:2 plan, so you can use them as a guideline to plan your own meals according to your personal needs and preferences.

SUNDAY

Meal one - morning-ish   about 220 calories

1 hard-cooked egg with 4 oz smoked salmon, coffee or tea

Meal two - evening-ish   about 275 calories

4 oz roasted chicken, skin removed, 1 cup kale salad, iced tea with lemon wedge

MONDAY

Meal one - morning-ish   about 204 calories

½ cup oatmeal with creamy peanut butter and ½ banana, coffee or tea

Meal two - evening-ish   about 275 calories

3 oz. seared flank steak; ½ cup sliced cherry tomatoes; iced tea

TUESDAY

Meal one - morning-ish   about 266 calories

Whole wheat toast with egg and ¼ avocado; 1 small or ½ large orange; coffee or tea

Meal two - evening-ish   about 240 calories

Stir-fry with chicken, snow peas, cabbage and carrots; ½ pear; sparkling water

WEDNESDAY

Meal one - morning-ish   about 180 calories

Strawberry banana yogurt smoothie; coffee or tea

Meal two - evening-ish   about 400 calories

1 cup stir-fried quinoa and vegetables; 1 cup mango cubes; iced tea

THURSDAY

Meal one - morning-ish   about 155 calories

Poached egg and Roma tomato slices on whole wheat toast, coffee or tea

Meal two - evening-ish   about 400 calories

Baked eggplant parmesan; tossed salad spritzed with olive oil and lemon juice; water

FRIDAY

Meal one - morning-ish   about 135 calories

½ cup lowfat cottage cheese; sliced apple with cinnamon; coffee or tea

Meal two - evening-ish   about 440 calories

Spaghetti squash with tomatoes, black olives, and feta cheese; 1 cup Caesar salad; iced tea

SATURDAY

Meal one   morning-ish   about   170 calories

Scrambled egg with low fat cheddar and salsa; coffee or tea

Meal two - evening-ish   about 360 calories

Grilled ahi tuna; 3 spears steamed broccoli; quinoa salad; iced tea

Keto/IF meal plan for non-fasting window

The meal plans in this section focus on the ketogenic way of dieting with high fat, moderate protein, and very low carbohydrates. The suggested meal plans are based on only two meals per day, but you can adjust that to suit your personal needs. There may be some days where just one sizeable meal will satisfy you, and other days when you need more than two meals to get you through the day. As long as your fasting/feeding schedule remains consistent, you'll be fine.

SUNDAY

Meal one: Eggs, bacon, sliced tomatoes

Meal two: Braised chicken thighs, mashed cauliflower, kale and brussel sprout salad

MONDAY

Meal one: Omelet with spinach and cheese

Meal two: Grilled steak, sautéed mushrooms, sliced tomatoes

TUESDAY

Meal one: Scrambled eggs with smoked salmon and avocado

Meal two: Ground beef patty with cheddar cheese and salsa, Mexican slaw

WEDNESDAY

Meal one: Tuna salad, celery sticks

Meal two: Turkey meatballs, sautéed spinach and mushrooms, side salad

THURSDAY

Meal one: Omelet with ham, cheese, onions, and peppers

Meal two: Grilled salmon and asparagus, avocado slices

FRIDAY

Meal one: Frittata with spinach, mushrooms, and parmesan

Meal two: Pork chop, charred green beans, keto Caesar salad

SATURDAY

Meal one: Cold roast beef slices, Swiss cheese cubes, avocado slices

Meal two: Pork and cabbage stir fry, cauliflower rice

A FINAL WORD

By now, you must have a pretty good idea of what intermittent fasting is and how it can help you lose weight and get healthy. One benefit that we haven't mentioned yet is how intermittent fasting can make your life simpler and relieve some of the stress of day to day living. Just think about it; if you are eating fewer meals, you're also spending less time cooking and shopping, and you're probably even saving yourself some money. And you have some extra time--the time that you would normally spend cooking and eating. You can use that time to be a little more productive at work or around the house, you can take up a new hobby, or you can just take some time to relax without feeling guilty.

Another benefit that we didn't mention is the way that intermittent fasting rejuvenates your palate, virtually waking it up. Going without food for a longer period of time gives your taste buds an opportunity to recharge and take on the next meal unhindered by leftover flavors and tired taste buds. Your next meal seems to burst with more flavors--the sweet, the sour, the salty, the bitter, and the umami--so that you enjoy the experience of eating more than you ever did before, not just because you missed the food, but because it actually tastes better. That's another reason to make sure you're choosing fresh, natural food for your meals.

For many people, intermittent fasting is far superior to old school dieting. Although it's difficult to deal with the hunger pangs in the beginning, they practically disappear as our hormones find their new rhythm, and our bodies adjust to not eating as frequently. Very few diets offer the multiple benefits of intermittent fasting: the weight loss, the improved health, the longer life, the mental clarity. The longer you maintain the practice of fasting, the more you will see the benefits. As research into intermittent fasting continues, as it must, it's entirely possible that even more benefits will be uncovered. There are not too many things in this world that have such an optimistic outlook.

ONE LAST THING... DID YOU ENJOY THE BOOK?

If so, then let me know by leaving a review on Amazon! Reviews are the lifeblood of independent authors. I would appreciate even a few words from you!

If you did not like the book, then please tell me! Email me at lizard.publishing@gmail.com and let me know what you didn't like. Perhaps I can change it. In today's world, a book doesn't have to be stagnant. It should be improved with time and feedback from readers like you. You can impact this book, and I welcome your feedback. Help me make this book better for everyone!

Made in the USA
Columbia, SC
07 June 2018